KNOWLEDGE GUIDE TO SCIATICA

Essential Manual To Proven Relief Methods, Pain Management Strategies, And Effective Exercises For Long Term Recovery

DR. AARON BRANUM

Copyright © 2024 BY DR. AARON BRANUM

All rights reserved. Except for brief quotations embodied in critical reviews and certain other noncommercial uses permitted by copyright law, no part of this publication may be reproduced, distributed, or transmitted in any form or by any means, Including photocopying, recording, or other electronic or mechanical methods, without the prior written permission of the publisher.

Disclaimer:

The data in this book, is solely meant to be informative and instructional.

This book is not intended to replace expert medical advice, diagnosis, or care. No medical, health, or other professional services are offered by the author, publisher, or any affiliated parties

Individual outcomes may differ in the practice of these therapies, which entail a variety of approaches and methodologies.

A one-on-one session with a trained or certified healthcare professional is still preferable. It is best to consult a trained healthcare provider before making any decisions regarding your health.

The author of this book is not affiliated with any specific website, product, or organization related to any of these therapies.

All reasonable measures have been taken by the author and publisher to guarantee the authenticity and dependability of the material contained in this book

Contents

CHAPTER ONE 15
ANATOMY AND FUNDAMENTALS 15
An Overview Of The Nervous System And Spine 15
Typical Reasons For Sciatic Nerve Pain 16
Recognizing The Differences Between Acute And Chronic Sciatica 18
The Value Of Good Body Mechanics And Posture 19

CHAPTER TWO 21
DIAGNOSIS AND ASSESSMENT 21
Medical Background Information And Physical Assessment 22
Exams To Diagnose Sciatica 23
Reading Imaging Studies (X-Rays, CT Scans, And Mris) 24
Evaluating Muscle Strength And Nerve Function 25
Cooperating With Medical Professionals To Make An Accurate Diagnosis 26

CHAPTER THREE 27

OPTIONS FOR TREATMENT 27
  Pain Relieving Drugs............................. 29
  Injectable Steroid Epidurals And Nerve Blocks 30
  Surgical Procedures For Serious Instances 31
  Alternative Medicine: Yoga, Chiropractic Treatment, And Acupuncture 33
CHAPTER FOUR 35
  CHANGES IN LIFESTYLE 35
  The Value Of Frequent Exercise And Flexibility 35
  Comfortable Positions For Standing, Sitting, And Lifting 36
  Weight Management And Its Impact On Sciatica 37
  Quitting Smoking And Its Role In Reducing Sciatic Pain 38
  Methods Of Stress Management For Pain Reduction 39
CHAPTER FIVE 41
  PREVENTIVE ACTIONS 41
  Techniques To Avoid Sciatica Recurrence . 42

Appropriate Body Mechanics For Everyday Tasks 44

Exercises To Support The Spine And Strengthen Core Muscles 45

Establishing A Comfortable Work Area 47

Including Relaxation And Mindfulness In Everyday Activities 48

CHAPTER SIX 51

SCIATICA MANAGEMENT AT WORK 51

Recognizing Your Situation 51

Applying Pain Reduction Methods 53

Talking To Employers About Your Situation 55

Providing Records Of Medical Treatment ... 56

Ergonomic Design Of Workspace 58

CHAPTER SEVEN 61

SETTING UP YOUR MONITOR 61

Setting Up Basic Workspace Items 61

Stretching And Taking Breaks During Work Hours 63

Using Tools And Assistive Devices 66

- Seeking Reasonable Adjustments In Compliance With Disability Laws 70
- Taking Part In Interactive Procedures 72

CHAPTER EIGHT 75
FAQS AND REGULAR QUESTIONS 75
- Can Sciatica Disappear By Itself? 75
- How Much Time Usually Does Sciatica Last? 76
- Is Surgery The Only Remedy In Extreme Situations? 77
- Can Sciatica Be Caused By Pregnancy? 78
- What Are Sciatica's Long-Term Consequences? 79

CHAPTER NINE 81
GOING AHEAD 81
- Developing A Customised Care Plan With Your Medical Staff 82
- Creating Reasonable Objectives For Pain Management And Rehabilitation 83
- Monitoring Development And Modifying Approaches As Required 84

Speaking Up For Yourself And Your Needs For Health 85

Adopting An Upbeat Attitude And Way Of Life For Long-Term Health 86

The Knowledge Guide to Sciatica is a glimmer of wisdom in the often bewildering and daunting world of health books. This thorough book dives deeply into the complex web of sciatica, providing readers with a profound understanding that gives them the confidence and clarity to walk their path to relief and recovery.

Fundamentally, this guide breaks down the enigmas and intricacies of sciatica to reveal its essence. It carefully breaks down the illness, from its causes to its symptoms, revealing the wide range of things that can set it off. Through a comprehensive examination of the origins and manifestations of sciatica, readers are provided with priceless insights into the significance of early identification, establishing the groundwork for prompt intervention and treatment.

Going deeper, the guide delves into the anatomy and fundamentals of sciatica, revealing the complex interplay between the spine and nerve system.

It clarifies the subtleties of the sciatic nerve and highlights how it helps the body communicate motor signals and feelings. With a detailed explanation of acute versus chronic sciatica, readers gain the insight necessary to handle the intricacies of their ailment.

Crucial chapters that lead readers through the maze of medical history, physical examination, and diagnostic tests are diagnosis and evaluation.

The book demystifies the diagnostic process, from interpreting imaging results to evaluating nerve activity, enabling people to work with healthcare practitioners successfully to achieve accurate diagnosis and individualized treatment programs.

A comprehensive and clear exploration of treatment choices is provided, ranging from conservative approaches to surgical techniques.

Readers are exposed to a range of treatment approaches with the goal of reducing pain and regaining function, from the healing properties of physical therapy to the therapeutic effectiveness of epidural steroid injections.

Changes in lifestyle take center stage, highlighting the significant influence of daily routines on sciatic health. Readers are guided towards revolutionary lifestyle adjustments that act as the cornerstones of prevention and management, covering everything from the significance of consistent exercise to the subtleties of ergonomic posture.

Readers are given the tools necessary to negotiate the challenges of controlling sciatica in a variety of contexts as the journey progresses.

The book is a constant companion, providing comfort and direction at every turn, covering everything from employment adjustments to managing the psychological effects of chronic pain.

Frequently asked questions and common concerns are handled with compassion and knowledge, debunking urban legends and false beliefs with data-driven analysis.

Readers can make educated judgments regarding their health by knowing everything from the typical course of sciatica to its long-term effects and implications for pregnancy.

The manual encourages users to choose their own route to recovery and well-being going ahead. With a customized treatment plan in place and a helpful healthcare staff at their side, people feel encouraged to speak up for themselves and adopt an optimistic outlook that opens the door to a better tomorrow.

CHAPTER ONE

ANATOMY AND FUNDAMENTALS

An Overview Of The Nervous System And Spine

The spine is the main support structure in the human body, supporting vital organs and safeguarding the sensitive spinal cord.

It is composed of vertebrae, which are supported by ligaments and muscles and cushioned by discs. Via the vertebral canal, the spinal cord, an extension of the brain, transmits and receives messages to and from the brain.

Knowledge of the Sciatic Nerve

The sciatic nerve, which starts in the lower spine and runs down each leg, is the biggest nerve in the body.

It is essential for the communication of messages from the brain to the lower limbs. When this nerve is compressed or irritated, it can cause sciatica or sciatic nerve pain. Symptoms along the nerve's route may include tingling, numbness, or intense pain.

Typical Reasons For Sciatic Nerve Pain

A ruptured disc

The sciatic nerve roots may be compressed by a herniated disc, also referred to as a slipped or ruptured disc, which can result in pain and discomfort.

This is frequently caused by rapid trauma or wear and tear, which causes the disc's interior gel-like fluid to leak out and irritate surrounding nerves.

a spinal stenosis

The disease known as spinal stenosis is characterized by spinal canal narrowing, which puts pressure on the sciatic nerve as well as the spinal cord.

Sciatica symptoms can result from this narrowing for a variety of reasons, including aging, arthritis, or congenital disorders.

The Piriformis Syndrome

The sciatic nerve can occasionally get irritated or compressed when it travels beneath the piriformis muscle in the buttocks.

Known medically as piriformis syndrome, this disorder causes pain and other symptoms akin to sciatica and may be brought on by overuse, injury, or spasms in the muscles.

Recognizing The Differences Between Acute And Chronic Sciatica

Severe Sciatica

Acute sciatica is the term used to describe quick onset pain and discomfort along the sciatic nerve, frequently brought on by a particular trauma or injury. Sharp, shooting pain, tingling, or numbness are some symptoms; these usually affect one side of the body. Although acute sciatica can be quite painful, it normally goes away with the right therapy and self-management techniques.

Prolonged sciatica

Contrarily, chronic sciatica is characterized by recurrent or persistent pain along the sciatic nerve that can endure for several weeks, months, or even years.

It could be brought on by underlying illnesses such as spinal arthritis or degenerative disc degeneration.

The symptoms of chronic sciatica can greatly affect daily functioning, necessitating long-term management techniques to reduce pain and enhance quality of life.

The Value Of Good Body Mechanics And Posture

It is essential to maintain good body mechanics and posture in order to avoid and treat sciatic nerve discomfort.

Slouching or prolonged sitting can lead to poor posture, which puts undue strain on the spine and aggravates sciatica symptoms.

Proper posture and the use of ergonomic furniture and equipment can help people with sciatic nerve pain by lessening the strain on their spines.

Furthermore, strengthening the muscles that support the spine and promoting general spinal health can be achieved by including regular exercise, stretching, and proper lifting techniques in everyday activities.

CHAPTER TWO

DIAGNOSIS AND ASSESSMENT

In order to precisely determine the underlying cause of the symptoms, a thorough evaluation approach is required for the diagnosis of sciatica.

A comprehensive medical history and physical examination are usually the first steps. The healthcare professional will ask about the beginning, duration, and nature of the pain, along with any aggravating or mitigating variables, during the medical history.

Inquiries on any past injuries or illnesses that might have contributed to the symptoms will also be made.

Medical Background Information And Physical Assessment

Healthcare professionals can better understand a patient's general health and any potential risk factors for sciatica by reviewing a thorough medical history.

This could include past medical issues like diabetes or arthritis, as well as surgeries and injuries.

The medical professional will measure a number of things during the physical examination, such as feeling, reflexes, and range of motion in the afflicted area.

In order to replicate the patient's symptoms and determine any underlying causes, such as spinal stenosis or herniated discs, they might also carry out particular maneuvers.

Exams To Diagnose Sciatica

To further assess the cause of sciatica, diagnostic testing may be conducted in addition to the medical history and physical examination.

Imaging procedures that offer fine-grained images of the spine and adjacent structures, including MRIs, CT scans, or X-rays, can be part of these examinations.

These pictures aid in the diagnosis of anomalies such as spinal cord compression, bone spurs, and herniated discs.

To evaluate nerve function and muscle activity, further tests such as nerve conduction studies or electromyography (EMG) may be carried out.

Reading Imaging Studies (X-Rays, CT Scans, And Mris)

One of the most important steps in diagnosing sciatica is interpreting imaging results. By obtaining precise images of the soft tissues of the spine through magnetic resonance imaging (MRI) scans, medical professionals can detect anomalies such as compressed nerve fibers, herniated discs, and more.

Computed tomography (CT) scans produce detailed pictures of the bone structures in the spine by using X-rays to create cross-sectional images.

Moreover, X-rays can be utilized to evaluate the spine's alignment and spot any fractures or degenerative changes.

Evaluating Muscle Strength And Nerve Function

Healthcare professionals can assess the degree of nerve injury and uncover any underlying neurological problems by measuring muscular strength and nerve function.

Studies on nerve conduction quantify the strength and speed of electrical signals that pass through nerves, whereas electromyography (EMG) evaluates how muscles contract in response to nerve stimulation.

These examinations can assist in distinguishing sciatica from other illnesses including muscular strain or peripheral neuropathy.

Cooperating With Medical Professionals To Make An Accurate Diagnosis

Getting a precise sciatica diagnosis requires cooperation with medical professionals. Open communication on symptoms, medical history, and concerns should be fostered between patients.

In order to create a customized treatment plan, medical professionals can then carry out a comprehensive evaluation, request the necessary tests, and evaluate the findings. Patients and medical professionals can enhance the quality of life and manage sciatica more successfully when they collaborate.

CHAPTER THREE
OPTIONS FOR TREATMENT

Although sciatica can be an uncomfortable and chronic ailment, there are a number of treatment options that can help control symptoms and encourage recovery.

People can make more educated judgments regarding their healthcare journey if they are aware of these options.

Conservative measures include physical therapy, ice, heat, and rest.

The first line of treatment for sciatica symptoms is frequently conservative measures. Resting eases the load on the injured area and gives the body time to recuperate.

By numbing the area and reducing inflammation, applying ice packs can temporarily ease discomfort. On the other hand, heat therapy helps ease discomfort, relax muscles, and increase blood flow.

Physical therapy is essential for managing sciatica because it emphasizes stretches and exercises that increase flexibility and strengthen the muscles that support the spine.

When a patient's condition improves, a physical therapist can create a regimen that is specifically tailored to meet their needs and advance gradually.

By implementing these conservative treatments into daily life, people with sciatica can greatly decrease the frequency and intensity of flare-ups, regain their mobility, and return to their regular activities.

Pain Relieving Drugs

Medication may be used to treat sciatica-related pain and inflammation when conservative approaches are insufficient. Pain and swelling can be lessened with the use of nonsteroidal anti-inflammatory medicines (NSAIDs), such as naproxen or ibuprofen.

Muscle relaxants may be recommended for more severe pain in order to reduce spasms and increase the range of motion. Antidepressants and anticonvulsants can influence how the brain interprets pain signals, which is why they are sometimes prescribed to treat chronic pain.

The best prescription schedule should be chosen in close consultation with a healthcare professional, taking into account each patient's unique needs and medical background.

Furthermore, people ought to be aware of possible adverse reactions and communicate any worries to their healthcare professionals.

Injectable Steroid Epidurals And Nerve Blocks

For those with persistent sciatica pain, interventional therapies such as nerve blocks and epidural steroid injections can offer focused relief. A corticosteroid drug is administered directly into the epidural area around the spinal nerves during an epidural steroid injection, which reduces inflammation and relieves pain.

In a similar vein, nerve blocks entail the temporary blocking of pain signals by injecting a local anesthetic close to the afflicted nerve or nerves. Through this surgery, people may experience instant alleviation and be better able to engage in physical therapy or other forms of rehabilitation.

Even though these treatments can provide a great deal of relief, they are usually saved for situations in which more conventional therapies have failed and the symptoms still don't go away.

Surgical Procedures For Serious Instances

Surgical intervention may be considered in severe cases of sciatica when conservative therapies and interventional procedures are ineffective in relieving the condition.

By removing bone spurs or herniated discs that are compressing the nerves, surgeons hope to relieve pressure on the afflicted nerve roots.

Discectomy, laminectomy, and spinal fusion are common surgical treatments for sciatica; each is designed to address a certain underlying cause of nerve compression. Modern surgical methods, like minimally invasive procedures, have helped many patients recover faster and have better results.

Surgery is typically only advised in cases where all non-invasive and conservative therapies have failed and the symptoms have a severe negative influence on one's mobility or quality of life.

Before undergoing surgery, patients should carefully weigh the advantages and disadvantages of the procedure with their healthcare professional and look into other choices.

Alternative Medicine: Yoga, Chiropractic Treatment, And Acupuncture

Alternative therapies can provide supplementary methods for treating sciatica symptoms and enhancing general health in addition to standard medical care. Tiny needles are inserted into particular bodily locations during the ancient Chinese art of acupuncture in order to promote energy flow and reduce pain.

The main goals of chiropractic care are to relieve nerve pressure and restore normal alignment of the spine through manipulation and adjustments. Chiropractors treat spinal abnormalities and misalignments to help patients with sciatica feel less pain and move more freely.

Yoga encourages strength, flexibility, and relaxation through a combination of physical postures, breathing techniques, and meditation. Certain yoga positions can help with sciatica symptoms by focusing on the muscles that support the spine, enhancing posture, and releasing stress.

Working with licensed professionals who have treated patients with comparable conditions is crucial when integrating alternative therapies into a sciatica management plan. In order to guarantee an all-encompassing and well-coordinated approach to care, people should also have open lines of communication with their medical professionals.

CHAPTER FOUR

CHANGES IN LIFESTYLE

Living with sciatica frequently requires modifying one's lifestyle to reduce pain and accelerate recovery.

These adjustments cover a wide range of day-to-day activities, such as exercise, posture, controlling weight, and stress management.

People can improve their general well-being and lessen the effects of sciatic pain by consciously changing.

The Value Of Frequent Exercise And Flexibility

The key to treating sciatica is to stretch and exercise on a daily basis. These exercises strengthen muscles, increase range of motion, and reduce stress in the afflicted area.

Walking, swimming, and yoga are examples of low-impact workouts that can successfully target the muscles around the sciatic nerve without making the pain worse.

Stretches that target the hamstrings, lower back, and hips can also help relieve pain and stop flare-ups in the future.

Comfortable Positions For Standing, Sitting, And Lifting

It's critical for people with sciatica to maintain good posture and body mechanics. When it comes to standing for extended periods of time, lifting weights, or sitting at a desk, ergonomics can reduce sciatic nerve pressure and associated discomfort.

Lower back strain and sciatic pain can be considerably reduced by using supportive chairs with lumbar support, modifying workstation heights to encourage neutral spine posture, and using safe lifting practices.

Weight Management And Its Impact On Sciatica

Excess weight can cause sciatic pain by exerting additional strain on the spine and associated muscles. Therefore, keeping a healthy weight through balanced nutrition and frequent exercise is vital for managing symptoms.

By choosing a nutritious diet rich in fruits, vegetables, lean meats, and whole grains, individuals can promote their general health and minimize inflammation in the body.

Additionally, integrating regular physical exercise can aid with weight control and strengthen muscles to support the spine, easing the strain on the sciatic nerve.

Quitting Smoking And Its Role In Reducing Sciatic Pain

Smoking has been related to an increased chance of getting sciatica and aggravating current symptoms.

Cigarette smoke contains compounds like nicotine that can impede blood flow to the spine, resulting in less oxygen and nutrients reaching the affected area.

Furthermore, smoking can aggravate sciatic pain over time by causing tissue damage and inflammation.

Therefore, giving up smoking is essential for anyone looking for sciatica relief because it can enhance spinal health overall, lower inflammation, and increase circulation.

Methods Of Stress Management For Pain Reduction

High levels of stress are frequently associated with chronic pain problems like sciatica, which can worsen symptoms and lower overall quality of life.

By putting stress management strategies into practice, people can enhance their general well-being and learn to manage pain more skillfully.

Techniques such as progressive muscle relaxation, deep breathing exercises, meditation, and guided imagery can ease the mental anguish brought on by chronic pain while also encouraging relaxation and reducing tenseness in the muscles.

Taking part in pleasant activities, interacting with people who are supportive, and obtaining professional counseling or therapy can all help to improve stress resilience and cultivate a positive outlook on treating sciatica.

CHAPTER FIVE

PREVENTIVE ACTIONS

A preventive approach can make a big difference in preventing sciatica. Keeping a healthy weight is one of the basic preventive strategies. Carrying too much weight might increase sciatic nerve discomfort and cause needless strain on your spine. You can lose those excess pounds and de-stress by sticking to a healthy diet and regular exercise schedule.

Keeping proper posture is another important protective step. Inadequate posture may play a role in compressing the sciatic nerve, resulting in pain and discomfort. Maintaining the appropriate alignment of your spine is crucial whether you're sitting, standing, or walking. This can be accomplished by engaging in mindfulness exercises and monitoring how your body is positioned throughout the day.

Moreover, sciatica can be avoided by avoiding extended standing or sitting. Prolonged sitting can compress the sciatic nerve, while prolonged standing can strain the muscles that surround the spine. In order to ease this pressure and preserve spinal health, it's imperative that you take regular breaks and exercise throughout your daily schedule.

Techniques To Avoid Sciatica Recurrence

Preventing the recurrence of sciatica is just as crucial as preventing its original occurrence. Including low-impact workouts in your regular regimen is one smart move. Engaging in physical activities like yoga, swimming, or walking might help strengthen the muscles that support your spine and lower your chance of flare-ups in the future.

Steering clear of activities that aggravate sciatic nerve pain is another important tactic. This could involve doing a lot of heavy lifting, moving quickly, or spending a lot of time sitting or standing awkwardly. You can reduce the chance that sciatica will repeat by paying attention to your body and avoiding painful activities.

Keeping up a healthy lifestyle can also be very helpful in preventing the recurrence of sciatica. This entails controlling stress levels, maintaining a healthy diet, and obtaining adequate sleep. By maintaining good overall health, you can lower the likelihood of sciatic nerve irritation by supporting normal nerve function and reducing inflammation in the body.

Appropriate Body Mechanics For Everyday Tasks

Maintaining good body mechanics is crucial to avoiding sciatica and putting the least amount of tension on the spine. These tips can help protect your back whether you're sitting at your computer, picking up something, or moving large goods.

Always remember to keep your back straight and bend your knees when lifting anything. When lifting, try not to twist your spine since this might put a strain on your muscles and compress your sciatic nerve. Instead, to lessen the tension on your back, power the lift with your leg muscles and keep the object close to your body.

Make careful to keep your shoulders relaxed and your spine in alignment when you're seated. Steer clear of slouching and relieve pressure on the sciatic nerve by using a chair that provides adequate lumbar support. To avoid stiffness and relieve strain on the spine, take frequent breaks to stand up, stretch, and move about.

Exercises To Support The Spine And Strengthen Core Muscles

For the spine to be supported and sciatica to be avoided, strengthening the core muscles is essential. Exercises for the back, pelvic, and abdominal muscles can assist increase stability and lower the chance of injury.

The plank is a useful exercise to strengthen the core. Starting in a push-up posture, place your hands just beneath your shoulders and align your body in a straight line from your head to your heels to begin a plank. As long as you can, maintain this posture while using your core muscles. Repeat multiple times to gradually increase your strength.

The bridge is another useful practice. With your feet flat on the ground and your knees bent, lie on your back.

Raise your hips off the floor so that your shoulders and knees are in a straight line. After a little period of holding this posture, drop your hips once more. To target the muscles in your lower back and buttocks, repeat multiple times.

By including these exercises in your normal training regimen, you can lessen your chance of developing sciatica and strengthen the muscles that support your spine.

Establishing A Comfortable Work Area

A lot of people spend a lot of time at a desk, which can aggravate sciatic nerve discomfort and lead to bad posture.

Establishing an ergonomic workstation is crucial for maintaining spinal health and avoiding pain.

To begin with, make sure your chair and workstation are at the proper height to encourage proper posture. When sitting, your knees should be 90 degrees from the floor and your feet should be flat on the ground.

If you want to relieve strain on your lower back and preserve the natural curve of your spine, use a chair with adjustable lumbar support.

Put your computer monitor at eye level as well to avoid putting undue pressure on your shoulders and neck.

To lessen the strain on your arms and shoulders and to avoid reaching, keep your keyboard and mouse near your body. Frequent breaks for stretching and movement can also help reduce pressure on the spine and avoid stiffness.

Including Relaxation And Mindfulness In Everyday Activities

Controlling stress is critical to avoiding sciatica and enhancing general health. Sciatic nerve discomfort may worsen as a result of chronic stress-related inflammation and tense muscles.

You can lessen stress and release tension in your body by incorporating mindfulness and relaxation practices into your everyday routine.

Exercises including deep breathing are one useful method. Throughout the day, set aside some time to concentrate on your breathing, taking slow, deep breaths with your nose and releasing them through your mouth. This has the potential to ease muscle tension and trigger the body's relaxation response.

Progressive muscular relaxation is another useful technique. Beginning at your toes and working your way up to your head, begin by tensing and then relaxing each muscle group in your body.

This can relieve strain on the sciatic nerve by encouraging relaxation and lowering general muscle tension.

Including practices like tai chi, yoga, or meditation in your everyday routine can also aid in promoting relaxation and lowering stress levels. These exercises assist optimal nerve activity, lessen the risk of sciatica flare-ups, and enhance your emotional well-being.

CHAPTER SIX

SCIATICA MANAGEMENT AT WORK

Recognizing Your Situation

Understanding your problem is the first step towards managing sciatica at work. Sciatica is a pain that radiates down each leg from your lower back along the sciatic nerve. It is a sign of an underlying medical disease, such as a herniated disc. You can more effectively manage your sciatic pain during working hours if you are aware of its triggers and patterns.

Putting Comfort First

Comfort is a top priority when it comes to controlling sciatica at work. Make sure that everything in your workspace—desk, chair, and computer configuration—is ergonomically built to support your spine and lessen the strain on your sciatic nerve. Getting a lumbar support chair and altering the height of your desk are two important steps you may take to lessen discomfort when working long hours.

Including Movement

It's critical to include mobility in your workday as sciatic discomfort can worsen with prolonged sitting. Make sure you take regular breaks to move about, stretch, and stand up to relieve pressure on your sciatic nerve and lower back. You can set reminders to remind you to shift postures frequently and to avoid lingering in one place for extended periods of time.

Maintaining Correct Posture

Keeping your posture correct is crucial to controlling sciatica at work. Avoid hunching over or slanting forward when sitting; instead, maintain a straight back and relaxed shoulders. To maintain your knees at hip level and your feet supported, use a footrest. Throughout the day, try to alternate between standing and sitting at a standing desk, if at all possible.

Applying Pain Reduction Methods

When sciatic pain starts, include pain management practices in your work routine to help relieve it.

To relieve tension and calm tight muscles, engage in deep breathing exercises. To relieve aching areas, apply heat or cold therapy using an ice pack or heating pad. Topical lotions or over-the-counter painkillers may also offer momentary relief.

Speaking with Coworkers

An environment at work that is supportive of sciatica management can be established via open communication with your coworkers. Tell them about your condition and any modifications you might require to carry out your duties efficiently. Encourage empathy and understanding among coworkers, and don't be afraid to ask for help when you need it.

Getting Expert Assistance

If self-management measures don't considerably improve your sciatica-related work limitations, get expert assistance. Speak with a physical therapist or your healthcare practitioner to create a customized treatment plan that meets your needs. They can offer advice on how to better manage your sciatica at work through exercises, ergonomic changes, and other interventions.

Talking To Employers About Your Situation

Teaching Your Employer

It's important to educate your employer about your sciatica in order to discuss it with them. Describe sciatica, its symptoms, and the ways in which it interferes with your professional life. Assist your employer in comprehending the obstacles you encounter and the modifications that can facilitate your efficient execution of job responsibilities.

Making an Accommodation Request

Make proactive requests for accommodations so you can control your sciatica at work. This could entail making changes to your workstation, such as adding ergonomic equipment or modifying your schedule to make time for stretches and breaks. Clearly state what you require and how these modifications will help the business and you.

Providing Records Of Medical Treatment

You can bolster your accommodation request with official medical records from your physician. Your diagnosis, treatment strategy, and any limits or limitations pertaining to your sciatica should all be included in this paperwork. Clear and comprehensive paperwork makes the accommodation process easier for your employer to handle and helps them recognize the validity of your requests.

Working Together to Find Solutions

Take a cooperative approach when speaking with your boss to identify solutions that benefit both of you. Be receptive to advice and prepared to make concessions when needed. Discuss innovative ways to meet your demands while preserving efficiency and production, such as job reorganization or telecommuting choices.

Resolving Issues

Be ready to respond to any queries or worries your employer may have about your accommodations and condition. Reassure them that you are still dedicated to doing your job duties as effectively as possible and that the accommodations you have asked for will assist you in reaching this objective. Assure them that you are taking proactive steps to manage your sciatica and are looking for ways to reduce how much it affects your ability to do your job.

Continuation

Following up with your employer to make sure accommodations are being implemented properly and to resolve any potential problems should be done on a frequent basis. Keep lines of communication open on your health and any modifications to your requirements or capabilities. By remaining involved, you can collaborate to establish a welcoming and inclusive workplace.

Ergonomic Design Of Workspace

Selecting the Ideal Chair

Making an ergonomic chair choice is essential for a sciatica-friendly workstation configuration. Seek for a chair with armrests, lumbar support, and a seat height that can be adjusted. In order to support your hips and lower back without placing pressure on your sciatic nerve, the seat should be firm and offer enough padding.

Changing the Desk Height

Your back and sciatic nerve can experience less strain when your desk is at the right height. When typing or writing, make sure your desk is at a comfortable height so your arms can rest there at a 90-degree angle. Use a keyboard tray or adjustable risers to raise or lower your desk to the perfect height.

CHAPTER SEVEN

SETTING UP YOUR MONITOR

To maintain proper posture and lessen shoulder and neck strain, place your computer monitor squarely in front of you at eye level. To avoid eye strain, change the font size and brightness. If needed, utilize an anti-glare screen. To prevent squinting or bending forward, hold the display at arm's length distance.

Setting Up Basic Workspace Items

Keep the necessities of your workstation close at hand to reduce the amount of time you spend reaching or bending, which can exacerbate sciatic pain. To save needless strain, keep commonly used goods like pens, notebooks, and office supplies close at hand. For an efficient workstation that is free of clutter, use desk organizers or drawers.

Establishing a Cosy Ambience

Add ergonomic equipment to your desk to increase comfort and productivity. To support your feet and ease the strain on your lower back, think about utilizing a footrest. Add a cushion or lumbar roll for extra support, particularly if the lumbar support on your chair is inadequate. Add plants or pictures to your desk to make it uniquely yours and to help you decompress.

Taking Intermittent Rests

Managing sciatica at work requires regular breaks, regardless of how well-designed your workstation is. Set up recurring reminders to remind you to get up, stretch, and take short walks throughout the day. Include stretches that gently work your hamstrings, hips, and lower back to release tension and increase flexibility.

Stretching And Taking Breaks During Work Hours

The Value of Intervals

It's critical to take breaks during working hours in order to manage sciatica and avoid discomfort from prolonged sitting. By taking breaks, you can ease the strain on your sciatic nerve and lower back, enhance circulation, and lessen weariness and stiffness. To sustain productivity and well-being, plan brief pauses into your schedule for standing up, stretching, and moving about.

Stretching Activities

Stretching activities can help release stress and increase flexibility in your legs, hips, and lower back. Include them in your break routine. Perform mild stretches such as hamstring stretches, hip flexor stretches, and piriformis stretches to treat tight muscles contributing to sciatic discomfort. Throughout your break, hold each stretch for 15 to 30 seconds and then repeat a few times.

Move With Awareness

During breaks, engage in mindful exercise to lower tension and become more aware of your body. Use body awareness exercises, posture correction, and relaxation techniques like tai chi or yoga. To build a sense of peace and well-being, concentrate on taking deep breaths and intentionally releasing tension with each action.

Including Small Breaks

To avoid weariness and stiffness, include micro-breaks in your work schedule in addition to regular ones. Every thirty to sixty minutes, take a small break to stand up, stretch, and shift positions. To keep your focus and energy levels up throughout the day, take advantage of micro-breaks to rehydrate, realign your posture, and rearrange your workstation.

Making Use of Break Reminders

Remember to take regular breaks during your work, and use alarms or reminders. Set up technologies to remind you to take breaks at convenient times, such as desktop or smartphone apps. To maximize your break time and promote your general well-being, personalize reminders to include gentle instructions for mindfulness or stretching.

Establishing a Break Schedule

Create a regular break schedule that works well with your workday. Based on your workload and energy levels, choose the best times for breaks, and make self-care a priority by resolving to take regular pauses. Establish a specific room in your workstation for taking breaks so that you can stretch, engage in mindfulness exercises, or just unwind and replenish yourself before coming back to work feeling renewed and invigorated.

Using Tools And Assistive Devices

Chair with Ergonomics

Purchase an ergonomic chair made especially to support your spine and reduce sciatica while you sit for extended periods of time. Seek features that encourage good posture and lessen pressure on your sciatic nerve and lower back, such as lumbar support, adjustable seat height, and armrests. Try out several chair designs and configurations to determine which one best suits your needs in terms of comfort.

Cushion for Lumbar Support

Add a lumbar support cushion to your current chair to make it more comfortable and give your lower back more support. Select a cushion that encourages healthy spinal alignment and follows the natural curve of your spine. To ease sciatic pain and lessen the strain on your lumbar region as you sit, place the cushion at the small of your back.

Comfortable Mouse and Keyboard

To lessen the pressure on your wrists, arms, and shoulders when typing and using your computer, use an ergonomic keyboard and mouse. Seek for patterns that reduce repetitive motions that can aggravate sciatic discomfort and encourage a neutral wrist position. To keep your workstation pleasant and ergonomic, change the height and angle of your keyboard and mouse.

Converting Standing Desks

To switch between sitting and standing during the workday, think about utilizing a standing desk converter. You may quickly change the height of your office with a standing desk converter, which relieves the strain of prolonged sitting and improves posture and circulation. Try out several standing positions to determine the best ratio of standing to sitting for your comfort and output.

Foot Stool or Footrest

To ease the strain on your lower back and enhance circulation, support your feet and legs when seated with a footrest or footstool. Select a footrest that can be adjusted in height and angle to suit your personal preferences and encourage optimal ergonomic alignment. To promote a neutral sitting position and to pleasantly elevate your feet, place the footrest under your desk.

Transportable TENS Device

While at work, think about utilizing a portable TENS (transcutaneous electrical nerve stimulation) device to ease sciatic discomfort and encourage muscular relaxation.

Through electrodes applied to the skin, a TENS machine produces low-voltage electrical impulses that inhibit pain signals and promote the release of endorphins. As required, apply the TENS unit to target trouble spots and improve your general comfort and well-being at work.

Seeking Reasonable Adjustments In Compliance With Disability Laws

Comprehending Disability Laws

Learn about the laws and rules pertaining to disabilities that provide protection to those with impairments, especially those who suffer from sciatica.

These laws, which forbid discrimination against people with disabilities in the workplace and mandate that companies make reasonable accommodations for qualified employees with disabilities, include the Americans with Disabilities Act (ADA) in the United States.

Finding Justifiable Modifications

Determine what kind of accommodations are reasonable and will allow you to continue performing your job duties in spite of your sciatica constraints.

Modifications to your workspace, changes to your work schedule or responsibilities, or the supply of assistive devices or tools are examples of reasonable accommodations.

To find suitable accommodations, take into account your unique needs and speak with your healthcare provider or a disability accommodation professional.

Making an Accommodation Request

Put your needs and how they relate to your sciatica in writing and ask your employer for reasonable accommodations.

To support your request, please submit supporting documents from your healthcare provider, such as a note from a physician or copies of your medical records.

Provide detailed information on the accommodations you need and how they will help you carry out your job responsibilities.

Taking Part In Interactive Procedures

Find solutions that both you and your employer can agree on by participating in an interactive process to discuss possible adjustments.

Work with your employer to find modifications that will satisfy your demands and preserve the necessary aspects of your career.

To help with the accommodation process, be willing to give any information or paperwork as needed and be open to considering various solutions.

Putting an End to Conflicts

In the event that disagreements emerge over the provision of reasonable accommodations, try to resolve them through informal conversations, mediation, or formal grievance procedures in accordance with the policies and procedures of your workplace.

Address any issues you have with your employer and try to come to a solution that satisfies both your needs and the organization's legal requirements on disability discrimination in an open and courteous manner.

Fighting for Your Rights

As a person with a disability, you should fight for your rights by being aware of the laws and rules that apply to you, getting assistance from organizations that support people with disabilities or from legal resources, and speaking up for yourself when needed.

Work to create a culture that accepts and accommodates people with disabilities by educating yourself and others on the value of disability inclusion and equitable access in the workplace.

CHAPTER EIGHT

FAQS AND REGULAR QUESTIONS

Can Sciatica Disappear By Itself?

In many circumstances, sciatica can truly resolve itself. It frequently relies on the underlying reason why the sciatic nerve is being irritated.

For instance, if a herniated disc is the origin of the sciatica, the disc may eventually repair or shift, releasing pressure on the nerve.

Furthermore, conservative measures like rest, mild exercise, and over-the-counter painkillers may help some sciatica sufferers.

However, since some cases may need more rigorous treatment, it's crucial to keep an eye on symptoms and seek medical attention if they worsen or continue.

How Much Time Usually Does Sciatica Last?

Sciatica can last anywhere from a few months to several years, depending on a number of variables including the underlying reason, the intensity of the symptoms, and the patient's reaction to treatment.

When treated properly, sciatica can sometimes go away in a matter of days or weeks. Others, though, might experience it for several months or even longer.

Treatment must be administered with patience and consistency because pushing oneself too hard or hastening recovery can sometimes make symptoms worse.

Is Surgery The Only Remedy In Extreme Situations?

In cases of severe sciatica, surgery is not necessarily the first or only course of action.

The majority of sciatica patients can really be successfully treated with conservative measures including physical therapy, medication, and lifestyle changes.

By lowering sciatic nerve pressure, pain, and inflammation, these methods hope to aid in healing and alleviate symptoms.

If conservative measures are unable to relieve the condition or if there are particular indications—such as significant neurological deficits or structural problems—surgery may be necessary.

Before considering surgery, it is imperative to explore the advantages, disadvantages, and available options with a healthcare provider.

Can Sciatica Be Caused By Pregnancy?

Yes, some women may experience sciatica during pregnancy. Hormonal fluctuations, weight gain, and postural changes can all increase the pressure on the sciatic nerve during pregnancy. This can result in lower back, buttocks, and leg pain, tingling, and numbness.

Furthermore, when the uterus grows, it may compress the sciatic nerve, worsening the condition.

Thankfully, sciatica that develops during pregnancy usually goes away after delivery when the body reverts to its pre-pregnancy form. Prenatal exercises, good posture, and the use of supportive equipment are a few strategies that can assist reduce discomfort during pregnancy.

What Are Sciatica's Long-Term Consequences?

Sciatica can have different long-term impacts depending on a number of variables, including the underlying cause, the intensity of the symptoms, and how well the therapy works. People may occasionally have persistent pain or repeated sciatica attacks, particularly if the underlying cause is not sufficiently treated. Prolonged sciatica can greatly reduce quality of life by interfering with everyday activities, sleep, and mobility.

Persistent sciatic nerve pressure can also cause muscle weakness, loss of feeling, and over time, even abnormalities in gait or posture.

Therefore, in order to reduce the chance of long-term consequences, sciatica must be treated quickly and properly. In addition to preventing future flare-ups and promoting general spinal health, regular exercise, maintaining a healthy weight, and adopting proper posture and body mechanics can also be beneficial.

CHAPTER NINE
GOING AHEAD

After receiving a sciatica diagnosis, moving forward could be intimidating, but you can effectively manage the illness with the correct strategy and assistance. It's crucial to remember that sciatica is a manageable illness, and there are different treatment methods available to alleviate pain and increase mobility. By taking proactive steps and working closely with your healthcare team, you may recover control over your health and quality of life.

One key component of moving forward is educating oneself about sciatica. It might be helpful to you to make knowledgeable decisions regarding your care if you are aware of the causes, symptoms, and available treatments. It might also be helpful to learn about activities and lifestyle changes that can help control symptoms. By gaining information, you take an active role in your own healing process.

Developing A Customised Care Plan With Your Medical Staff

Developing a customized treatment program is necessary to effectively manage sciatica. Together, you and your healthcare team—which could consist of doctors, physical therapists, and pain specialists—will create a plan that is customized to meet your unique needs and objectives. A variety of therapies, including medicine, physical therapy, and complementary therapies like chiropractic or acupuncture, may be used in this regimen.

Your healthcare team will take into account a number of aspects while developing your treatment plan, such as the intensity of your symptoms, your general health, and your lifestyle. They will also consider any underlying medical disorders that could be causing your sciatica. You can make sure that your treatment plan is efficient and feasible for you by working closely with your healthcare team and actively engaging in the decision-making process.

Creating Reasonable Objectives For Pain Management And Rehabilitation

To successfully manage sciatica, realistic goal-setting is essential. Although it's normal to want pain and discomfort to go away right away, it's important to understand that rehabilitation takes time. Setting attainable goals will help you stay motivated and keep a good record of your progress.

Goal-setting requires being precise and quantifiable. It's also important to be realistic about what you can do in the timeframe you have given. For instance, instead of setting a generic aim like "reduce pain," you might set a precise objective like "increase walking distance without experiencing leg pain." Your medical team can assist you in defining objectives that are in line with your capabilities and constraints.

Monitoring Development And Modifying Approaches As Required

It's critical to monitor your development in order to assess the efficacy of your treatment plan and make any necessary modifications. To track your symptoms, activities, and any changes you notice over time, use a tracking tool or keep a notebook. This data can offer you and your healthcare team useful insights as well as assist you in spotting patterns and trends.

Be proactive in your communication with your healthcare team as you monitor your progress. Do not be afraid to seek advice if your symptoms are getting worse or if you are not getting the outcomes you had hoped for. To better manage your symptoms, your healthcare team can assist you in modifying your treatment strategy or looking into other possibilities.

Speaking Up For Yourself And Your Needs For Health

Taking care of your own needs is crucial when dealing with sciatica. Talk openly with your healthcare provider about your symptoms, worries, and preferred course of therapy. Since you are the one who knows your body the best, your advice is invaluable in creating a treatment strategy that suits you.

Furthermore, if you have any doubts about your diagnosis or recommended course of therapy, don't be afraid to get a second opinion. It's critical that you feel knowledgeable and secure in the choices you make for your health. You can make sure you get the attention and assistance you need to properly manage your sciatica by standing up for yourself.

Adopting An Upbeat Attitude And Way Of Life For Long-Term Health

For long-term well-being, adopting a positive outlook and way of life is crucial for those with sciatica. Even though controlling chronic pain might be difficult, keeping an optimistic mindset can enhance your quality of life in general. To help you relax and manage stress, try mindfulness exercises like deep breathing and meditation.

Apart from developing an optimistic outlook, concentrate on embracing wholesome living practices that enhance your overall health. This entails maintaining a healthy diet, exercising to the extent that is safe for you, getting enough sleep, abstaining from smoking, and limiting your alcohol intake. Over time, these lifestyle modifications may help you better manage the symptoms of sciatica and enhance your general health.

You can lessen the impact of symptoms on your everyday activities and enhance your quality of life by adopting a positive mentality and lifestyle and controlling your sciatica prophylactically. Keep in mind that you are not traveling alone and that there are resources available to assist you in overcoming the difficulties associated with having sciatica.

www.ingramcontent.com/pod-product-compliance
Lightning Source LLC
Chambersburg PA
CBHW071839210526
45479CB00001B/202